The Scoop on Cancer: A Medical Analysis on Cancer and its Treatments.

What is cancer?

In a healthy human body, cells die when necessary and divide and grow new ones when necessary. Cancer is the opposite of that. With cancer, cells don't die when they are supposed to and they divide and grow when they aren't supposed to. And this is what causes lumps and tumor- these unnecessary growths. This can cause all sorts of problems for the body. Cancer cells are resilient, in that they ignore the signals of apoptosis, the body's way of getting rid of old and damaged cells. They use the whole body to their advantage, even the immune system at times to work for the cancer. Cancer comes from the DNA in the the cells being mutated which may be genetics inherited but mainly it is from a variety of environmental factors such as ultraviolet rays or smoking, and the like.

The cure-

The cure seems simple then, change the DNA and genetics back to normal functionality. The problem is that there are so many cells dividing and spreading with this cancer DNA, that it is very hard to chase the cancer. This is why Dr. Perter Glidden explained that there are flaws to chemotherapy and many other treatments mainly used today. For they are using reduction treatments removing as many cancer cells as they can and taking some of the good cells with them. But that doesn't cure the core of the disease, when the cancer is holistic and needs to be treated as such. We will now go into this in more detail.

What is chemotherapy?

Dr. Peter Glidden in an interview discusses a study done in 1994, a twelve year medi-analysis published in The Journal of Clinical Oncology of adults who had cancer and were treated with chemotherapy. 97% of the chemotherapy treatments did not work. He gave an analogy if Ford came out with a car that failed 97% of the time, would it still be in business? But that is the point. America has lost the war on cancer in Dr. Peter and many others opinion because it is a "for profit" disease. Dr. Peter explains that the chemotherapeutic drugs are sold to doctors for one price and sold to the patient for estimated double that price. This is why chemotherapy has kept its main status. Dr. Peter has a book called "The MD Emperor has No Clothes" where you can read more of his findings.

Why chemotherapy mainly does not work-

Chemotherapy is short term for "chemical therapy". But that is such a vague terminology-like what kind of chemicals are used, and why is that part so underplayed?

How chemotherapy began-

In World War One the use of mustard gas as a weapon caused thousands and thousands of deaths. So when World War Two came about, Dr. Louis Goodman and Dr. Alfred Gilman of Yale University looked into cures for this weapon of destruction. The doctors noticed that the victims exposed to mustard gas had low counts of white blood cells. They hypothesized that if the mustard gas could be used to kill good white blood cells, it could kill the bad cells as well. They noticed it worked, although the patient had to come back for more chemo afterwards.And yes, nowadays part of chemo is still used from mustard gas, nitrogen mustard, as well as over one-hundred other chemicals.

The problem with this treatment-

As explained above, the death of both the bad cells and the good cells are involved with this kind of treatment. This is what makes people's hair fall out and feel weak- because chemotherapy is actually killing them and their cells. The hope is that when they regenerate, the only cells that will regenerate will be cancer free. And 3% of the time it works, but that is not good enough.

Cancer.org explains how some of the chemicals used in chemotherapy work very clearly:

Many of the chemicals in chemotherapy are alkylating agents, meaning they "keep the cell from reproducing by damaging the DNA". (12) They even say there that the concern is that the cancer will just come back even years down the line. And why is that? Because chemotherapy is just pushing it away temporarily. The same risk of cancer coming back is from another part in chemo they use, called Topoisomerase II inhibitors. Then they have the anti-tumor group of chemotherapy which sounds perfect from the name. But these also effect the body and DNA very strongly and can permanently damage people's hearts so have "lifetime limits" to be administered on how long they will give it to a patient. The mitotic inhibitors part of chemotherapy can cause nerve damage. Chemotherapy will usually be a mix of all these chemicals, so no wonder the people look and feel so sick from being on chemo.

The other mainstream treatments-

It's possible for radiation, homotherapy, and the like to kill cancer. Their attempt is to target the cancer cells but good cells nearby are also damaged. And yet, these therapies could easily leave some cancer cells still alive, which may eventually grow back. Not to mention that these treatments can cause secondary cancers and other problems down the line from the radiations and chemicals used in them.

Radiation- uses high energy radiation such as x-rays and gamma rays to kill the cancer cells.

-Side effects could be fatigue, long term serious skin problems, and long term effects such as the damages of being exposed to radiation ie a secondary cancer. It also takes months to do, leaving patients exhausted.

Hormone Therapy-

This is the treatment of slowing down hormones in the place where the cancer is, ie in the breast, prostate, or uterine. But the change of hormones can have a very long list of side effects from hot flashes to blood clots and seizuring. It is similar to all the other reduction treatments in that they are not attacking the problem directly.

Immunotherapy: Immunotherapy is the administration of living organisms to stimulate the immune response, which often leaves the patient with flu-like symptoms.(11)

Immunotherapy can take 3-5 years to be administered which is crazy long. It can affect the good cells with the bad like all these other treatments. Also side effects can include sensitive skin reactions such as blistering and mouth sores.

Surgery- when the cancer has not spread and is all contained in specific spot, surgery could work for that and remove let's say a tumor. Even so, some of the good tissues in the body are removed along with the bad ones, and there is no saying the surgery will remove all the cancer cells.

Targeted therapy-

According to BreastCancer.org, targeted therapies are treatments that single out specific characteristics of cancer cells, such as a protein that allows the cancer cells to grow in a rapid or abnormal way.

But Targeted therapy still does not hit the cancer directly. It is just looking for cells that have characteristics that would seem to be cancer and it is still like an estimation game which is not effective enough.

So let's talk about some more effective treatments:

1. CICD- Caspase-Independent Cell Death

"Conventional anti-cancer treatments work by apoptosis, a kind of programmed cell death where cells effectively get ordered to kill themselves off, via proteins called caspases.

It's how chemotherapy works, for example, and it can work well – but there are caveats.

These therapies can miss some of their targets, which means cancer cells don't get eliminated and the tumours have a better chance of coming back, and can also be damaging to healthy cells, as anyone who's been through chemotherapy will tell you.

Enter CICD, which takes on some of the mechanisms of apoptosis but takes caspases out of the equation. When cells are killed off with CICD, the researchers found, they send a signal to the immune system that can then attack any remaining cancer cells.

It's a cleaner and hopefully safer way of taking a tumour out of a body – though it's worth emphasising that the treatment has only been tested on lab models so far. (1)

1. Gene therapy

A) The Bethesda Maryland based National Cancer Institute(NCI) is working on something amazing-

A tumor sample from Dr. Solit's patient underwent whole genome sequencing - meaning all genes within it were analyzed for mutations, or variations, in the repeat stretches of compounds called bases that make up the genetic code.

"She(the patient) had 17,000 mutations in her tumor that were not found in her normal cells," Solit said. After months of analyzing 140 mutations that were considered suspects, two of them - genes named TSC1 and NF2 - stood out.

"It was like, 'Wow,' that's why the patient was unique, and why even though Afinitor(a medicine) was generally disappointing (and did not work) in the bladder cancer trial, it was the right drug for her," Dr. Solit said. "It was the combination of both mutations that probably led to her complete response," especially the TSC1 mutation.

Zeroing in on the two genes among more than 20,000 human genes that make proteins would not have been possible even five years ago, Solit said. "Maybe we would have looked at one gene and if that didn't show anything we'd look at another. Now we can sequence the entire genome and look at every gene, every needle in the haystack, at the same time."

By linking the TSC1 mutation to bladder cancer, Solit has discovered a new "biomarker," or suspected link, to the disease, while simultaneously identifying a possible appropriate drug for patients with any type of cancer who have that mutation. (13)

These kinds of treatments are really getting to the core of the genetics.

Another genetic treatment just recently was reviewed by CNN in late August of 2017 is something called Kymriah. The FDA approved it for treatment of leukemia. "Kymriah works by genetically modifying a patient's own cells so they can attack the cancer. Each dose of Kymriah contains a patient's own immune cells, which are sent to a lab to be genetically modified using a virus. This therapy, known as chimeric antigen receptor T-cell therapy, or CAR-T, gives the cells the ability to recognize and kill the source of the cancer." (14)

Now let's talk about some products that are found easily all over the world.

1. DCA (dichloroacetate sodium)

"DCA is a novel cancer agent because it doesn't directly kill cancer cells (the standard mechanism of most chemo agents, which renders their significant toxicity). Rather, it alters the unique metabolic features characteristic of cancer cells. Unlike healthy cells, cancer cells produce vast amounts of energy from glucose in a dysfunctional way. Cancer cells have the unique ability to over-express insulin receptors that transport glucose into the cancer cell. Here, via the process of glycolysis – the primary method of energy production for cancer cells – energy is produced from glucose without oxygen (even if oxygen is present)

This phenomenon was first observed by Nobel Prize laureate Otto Warburg in 1929 (known in science as the "Warburg Effect").

Rapidly growing tumor cells exhibit rates of glycolysis up to 200 times higher than those of healthy cells. In turn, the energy produced is used to fuel the growth and spread of cancer.

On the other hand, healthy cells do not primarily use glycolysis for energy production, because it's an inefficient way to produce energy. Instead, healthy cells use oxygen to produce energy from glucose in the mitochondria (the metabolic center) of the cell. The switch to glycolysis as an energy source occurs when cells of a tumor (either benign or pre-cancerous) become deprived of oxygen in their environment.

As a result, their mitochondria cannot work properly. These abnormal cells then 'switch off' their mitochondria. Mitochondria are essential to the process of inducing apoptosis (the process by which abnormal cells self-destruct). When cells switch off mitochondria, they develop "immortality" and can continue to divide.

Not all cells of a tumor develop ways to turn off their mitochondria and become immortal. Those that do, outlive the other cells in the tumor and these are the dominant cells that are responsible for the growth, spread (metastasis) and recurrence of disease. DCA specifically targets these dominant cells, producing the clinical observation that most individuals having their disease treated with DCA experience a partial or complete response to treatment and many have achieved stabilization of disease as well as cure.

In simpler terms, " It was observed that DCA would turn on natural apoptosis (cell death) in the cancerous cells of lab rats. It was also observed that DCA blocked the process by which glucose is used by cancer cells, thus removing their energy source and starving them." (7)

Although, There are some side effects noted:

Side effects to DCA are all **reversible**. With oral DCA, the most common side effects include: peripheral neuropathy (numbness in an area of the body, with or without associated nerve pain; experienced in 15% of patients), fatigue (15%) and confusion/reduced memory (15%). **IV DCA has fewer side effects and whatever side**

effects are experienced, are short-lived. No true allergy to DCA has ever been observed. (6)

They currently sell DCA on Amazon.com and some other places as well in powder and capsule form.

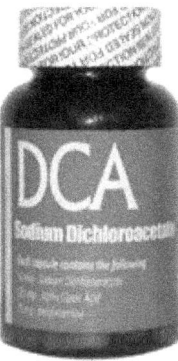

1. Blushwood Berry

'Scientists at QIMR Berghofer Medical Research Institute in Queensland have used an experimental drug produced from the seeds of the rainforest plant, Blushwood tree (Hylandia Dockrillii), which exclusively grows in far north Queensland, to cure solid cancer tumours in pre-clinical trials.

Already the drug has been used to successfully destroy or shrink tumours in pets and animals – including dogs, cats and horses and even Tasmanian Devils, while human trials are imminent.'

These results were discovered in an eight-year study led by Dr. Glen Boyle, from the QIMR Berghofer medical research institute in Brisbane. In 75% of cases, the cancer never returns. There were no side effects, and the compounds started working in five minutes, making cancerous melanoma and neck tumors disappear in a matter of days. (9)

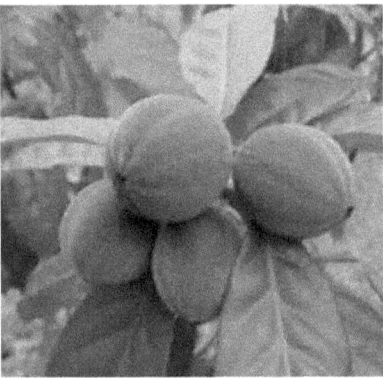

Like DCA, they need to do more research on the matter for blushwood berries, because these results are amazing.

1. B17 -This is a naturally occurring substance found in the pit of aprictots and in other foods such as the grain, millet. B17 does contain some cyanide, which is poisonous if you take it directly. But a moderate dose like b17 would not be as it is naturally occurring in many foods we eat. Other names for b17 is amygdalin or laetrile. It is illegal to be researched or obtain in the United States. There are Clinics for it in Mexico. In the U.S.,

they will say it's illegal because its ineffective and has cyanide in it. But when you do research on it you see the results are the opposite of that. There is a movie titled "A World Without Cancer" by G. Edward Griffin where he discusses animals who consume b17 foods did not develop cancer.

"What makes vitamin B17 so powerful is the fact that it is comprised of glucose and hydrogen cyanide. The way it actively destroys cancer cells is by the glucose 'injecting' itself into the cancer cell. Then the cyanide and benzaldahyde from the glucose create a targeted poison that kills the cancer cell. This natural form of chemotherapy was (and still is) considered controversial. Many medical professionals claim B17 is toxic. Well, the last time I checked, having cancer (in any form) is toxic in itself and causes death daily. The only thing B17 is toxic to is cancer cells and a corrupt government."
(10)

1. Cannabis- I suggest to take a look at each of these studies individually which you can view by clicking the links on the website put in bibliography #11

• A 1996 study discovered the protective effects of cannabinoids on the development of certain types of tumors. Cannabinoids were observed causing cell death, blocking cell growth, and preventing the development of the blood vessels tumors needed to grow — suggesting cannabinoids may be able to kill cancer cells while protecting normal cells.
• A series of studies on brain tumors conducted in 2003 proved CBD may make chemo more effective and increase the deaths of cancer cells without harming normal cells.

- A 2004 study on mice which showed cannabinoids protect against inflammation of the colon, thus reducing the risk of colon cancer and possibly aiding in its treatment.
- In 2011, the American Association for Cancer Research revealed CBD kills cells associated with breast cancerwhile having little to no effect on normal breast cells. When studied in mice, CBD reduced the growth, number, and spread of tumors.
- The National Institute of Healthpublished a study in 2011,Cell Death & Differentiation, that demonstrates THC andJWH-015 (a cannabinoid receptor), decreased the viability of liver cancer cells. Cannabinoids were also shown to inhibit tumor growth and the accumulation of fluid in the abdomen. These are significant findings as they may be helpful in the design of therapeutic strategies to manage liver cancer.
- A study published in February 2015 found rates of bladder cancer are 45% lower in cannabis users, compared to those who do not use it. (11)

A notable person who is worth looking up is Rick Simpson, who became famous for the oil named after him, "Rick Simpson Oil". He was a cancer patient whom the doctors had given up hope for. At home, he tried his own way of healing using cannabis oil and applying it on his skin. He noticed very fast results of the cancer going away and says the cannabis oil saved his life.

Cannabis Root- cannabis root has been used as a form of medicine documented as far back as the ancient Chinese in 2700 BCE, who wrote about its healing properties. The pentacyclic triterpene ketones in cannabis roots are also thought to cause apoptosis, or programmed cell death, in cancer cells. Though the research is minimal, cannabis roots may prove to possess effective cancer-fighting properties.(16)

It is interesting to note another root of a plant, that is also called a "weed", helped cure cancer.

7. The dandelion root-

"This root has been used medicinally since ancient times for its various health benefits. However, the most powerful benefit to come out of this common weed is something that medical researchers are super excited to have "discovered" – which is its potential to cure cancer! This potent root builds up blood and immune system- cures prostate, lung, and other cancers better than chemotherapy. According to Dr. Carolyn Hamm from the Windsor Regional Cancer Centre in Ontario, Canada, dandelion root extract was the only thing that helped with chronic myelomonocytic leukemia. This form of cancer typically affects older adults. John Di Carlo, who at the time was a 72-year old cancer patient at the hospital, was sent home to live out his final days after all efforts failed to treat his leukemia."

He told CBC News that he was advised to drink dandelion root tea as a last ditch effort. Perhaps it should have been the first option offered in his treatment plan, as his cancer went into remission only four months later! His doctors attributed this to the dandelion tea that he drank. Recent studies have shown that dandelion root extract can work very quickly on cancer cells, as was evidenced in Di Carlo's case. Within 48 hours of coming into contact with the extract, cancerous cells begin to disintegrate. The body happily replaces these with healthy new cells. Further studies have concluded that the extract also has anti-cancer benefits for other types of cancer, including breast, colon, prostate, liver, and lung cancer! Dandelion root tea may not taste as pleasant as other teas, but it's certainly more pleasant than living with the side effects of chemotherapy or radiation treatments. Traditional cancer therapies harm the immune system by killing all cells, even the healthy ones. Dandelion root has the opposite effect – it actually helps boost your immune system and only targets the unhealthy cells." (15)

Moringa Leaf- The Asian Pacific Journal of Cancer Prevention in 2003 published a study in which researchers examined skin tumor prevention following ingestion of moringa seedpod extracts in mice. Results showed a dramatic reduction in skin papillomas and suggested that M. oliefera has possible cancer preventing properties.

Another study conducted in 2006 reported that a molecule found in Moringa oleifera induced cell death in ovarian cancer cells grown in a lab. Based on these findings, researchers believe the plant has potential to treat this type cancer.

(20)

Food, vitamins, and Nutrition-

Ty Bollinger wrote a book called "The Truth about Cancer" that has some great tips. He discusses the mushroom and its healing abilities:

"Perhaps one of the most well-known medicinal mushroom in Asian healing arts is *Ganoderma lucidum*, or better known by its common name, reishi. The mushroom's bioactive molecules and polysaccharides have been shown to better activate natural killer (NK) cells reducing cancer metastasis. NK cells are lymphocytes that perform immunosurveillance within the body, constantly on the lookout for "immuno-alerters" signaling tumor presence." (2)

He discusses how the maitake mushroom has the same ability to activate the NK cells to defend against cancer.

Agaricus Blazei Murill- This mushroom made perhaps the biggest splash when a study jointly conducted by the Medical Department of Tokyo University, The National Cancer Center Laboratory, and Tokyo College of Pharmacy showed a complete recovery in 90% of guinea pigs injected with cancer cells (2)

Turkey Tail- The anti-viral properties of the turkey tail mushroom offer a unique opportunity to target oncoviruses (tumor virus) such as human papillomavirus leading to cervical cancer, hepatitis C leading to liver cancers, and others. For this mushroom, again studies are showing increased NK activity towards tumor detection and eradication. (2)

Cabbages- Cabbage helps prevent cancers of the breast, lung and colon, says Leonard Bjeldanes, a professor of food toxicology with the University of California at Berkeley. "The cancer rates come down as much as 40 percent when you go from low consumption of these vegetables to high consumption," he says. (17) A Finnish study found that the fermentation process involved in making sauerkraut from a cabbage produces several other cancer-fighting compounds, including ITCs, indoles, and sulforaphane. (18) Non-fermented cabbage though, will still be helpful in cancer treatment.

Tomatoes-
This juicy fruit is the best dietary source of lycopene, a carotenoid that gives tomatoes their red hue, Béliveau says. And that's good news, because lycopene was found to stop

endometrial cancer cell growth in a study in *Nutrition and Cancer*. Endometrial cancer causes nearly 8,000 deaths a year. (19) Lycopene is also found in watermelon.

Vitamin D-

In 2016 a landmark study in PLOS ONE found that women over 55 with blood concentrations of vitamin D higher than 40ng/ml, had a **67% lower risk** of cancer compared women with levels lower than 20ng/ml.

The researchers concluded that optimal levels for cancer prevention are between 40 and 60ng/ml, and that most cancers occur in people with vitamin D blood levels between 10 and 40ng/ml.

The study did not reveal whether supplementation or sun exposure was the best way to obtain vitamin D. However, the researchers concluded that vitamin D only starts protecting against cancer once you get you blood level up to 40 ng/ml. They noted that more health benefits were observed at higher levels of the vitamin. (3)

Vitamin K-Lab studies demonstrate tremendous potential for vitamin K in many cancer types.Vitamin K2 induces certain kinds of human leukemia cells to differentiate, or turn into normal white blood cells. In cells from certain brain tumors, in stomach cancer, and in colorectal cancer lines, vitamin K halts the reproductive cell cycle and induces apoptosis. Vitamin K also triggers a DNA-degrading protein that cancer cells normally suppress; thereby preventing tumor cells from repairing themselves effectively.

Lung cancers are notoriously aggressive and difficult to treat. In several different types of lung cancer, including **small cell, squamous cell,** and **adenocarcinomas,** vitamin K induces apoptosis through activation of a "suicide protein."Clinical trials of newer chemotherapy agents have been disappointing, but when vitamin K was added to one newer drug, *imatinib mesylate,* it rapidly suppressed growth in all lung cancer cell lines tested. Vitamin K exhibits similarly synergistic effects in bladder and liver cancers as well.

A unique mechanism of vitamin K's activity is so-called "oncosis," a form of stress-activated ischemic cell death to which tumor cells are particularly susceptible. Because of their high growth rate, tumor cells consume vast amounts of *glucose.* And because they can rapidly outgrow their blood supplies, that high metabolism means they use up oxygen rapidly, making them especially vulnerable to oxidant stress—much more so than the healthy tissues around them. Vitamin K targets tumor cells for destruction by stimulating oxidative stress, without toxicity to healthy tissues. (3)

Vitamin C-

Vitamin C, when administered in high doses by intravenous (I.V.) infusions, can kill cancer cells. Vitamin C interacts with iron and other metals to create hydrogen peroxide. In high concentrations, hydrogen peroxide damages the DNA and mitochondria of cancer cells and shuts down their energy supply and kills them outright.

Best of all — and unlike virtually all conventional chemotherapy drugs that destroy cancer cells — it is selectively toxic. No matter how high the concentration, Vitamin C does not harm healthy cells. (5)

Selenium- A Harvard study of more than 1,000 men with prostate cancer found those with the highest blood levels of selenium were 48 percent less likely to develop advanced disease over 13 years than men with the lowest levels. And a dramatic five-year study conducted at Cornell University and the University of Arizona showed that 200 micrograms of selenium daily—the amount in two unshelled Brazil nuts—resulted in 63 percent fewer prostate tumors, 58 percent fewer colorectal cancers, 46 percent fewer lung malignancies, and a 39 percent overall decrease in cancer deaths. (18)

Horoscope of Cancer The Crab-

The crab in Syrian is called the "sartano"- meaning to hold or scoop. This is named from the crab's claws, assumingely. The crab also shuffles when he walks and has his shell to hide in. Cancer makes you want to hide in your shell. Some of these amazing patients shuffle out of it, grab hold of that cancer, and throw it out the window.

A couple years ago I worked in Camp Sunrise Day Camp in Long Island, New York. It is a day camp for people who have went through cancer or going through it. Some of the campers and counselors have had cancer, or maybe it was somebody in their family that had it. In either case, everybody there held this deep value for life and that the sun will rise. This is why at the end of every camp day the camp would sing together, followed by some popsicles. This was another inspiration that led to this book being written.

FYI nobody paid me to endorse anything here, nor am I responsible for any of the treatments here. I only want you to see all the possibilities, and make up your own mind on the subject.

Bibliography:

1. https://www.sciencealert.com/scientists-find-a-new-way-to-attack-cancer-that-works-better-than-chemo

2. https://thetruthaboutcancer.com/medicinal-mushrooms-cancer/

3. https://www.chrisbeatcancer.com/vitamin-d-the-1-anti-cancer-vitamin.

4. http://www.lifeextension.com/magazine/2010/11/The-Remarkable-Anticancer-Properties-of-Vitamin-K/Page-01

5. https://www.cancertutor.com/vitaminc_ivc/

6. http://www.portmoodyhealth.com/cancer-centre/integrative-cancer-therapies/dca-dichloroacetate/

7. https://www.cancertutor.com/dca-treatment-for-cancer/

8. http://www.lifeextension.com/magazine/2010/11/The-Remarkable-Anticancer-Properties-of-Vitamin-K/Page-01

9. https://therenegadepharmacist.com/ebc-46-the-truth-about-the-australian-miracle-berry-extract-that-cures-cancer/

10. http://reset.me/story/vitamin-b-17-the-greatest-cover-up-in-the-history-of-cancer/

11. https://www.leafly.com/news/health/cannabis-and-cancer

12. https://www.cancer.org/treatment/treatments-and-side-effects/treatment-types/chemotherapy/how-chemotherapy-drugs-work.html

13. https://www.reuters.com/article/us-cancer-superresponders/looking-for-lessons-in-cancers-miracle-responders-idUSBRE98E07420130915

14. https://www.google.com/amp/s/amp.cnn.com/cnn/2017/08/30/health/fda-first-gene-therapy-leukemia/index.html

15. http://nativestuff.us/2017/06/scientists-find-root-that-kills-98-of-cancer-cells-in-only-48-hours/

16. https://www.learngreenflower.com/articles/154/10-things-you-never-knew-about-cannabis-roots

17. https://consumer.healthday.com/cancer-information-5/mis-cancer-news-102/fermenting-sauerkraut-foments-a-cancer-fighter-509840.html

18. https://www.google.com/amp/s/www.rd.com/health/conditions/10-foods-to-help-prevent-cancer/amp/

19.https://www.google.com/amp/amp.health.com/health/gallery/0,,20430736,00.html

20.https://www.google.com/amp/s/www.asbestos.com/blog/2014/10/24/moringa-leaves-alternative-cancer-treatment/amp/